Kidney Stone Diet Cookbook

A Complete Guide With Healthy and Delicious Recipes To Manage Kidney Problems

Table of Contents

Introduction 1

Types of Kidney Stones 2

Symptoms of Kidney Stone 3

What Causes Kidney Stones? 5

How are kidney stones diagnosed? 9

How to prevent kidney stones 12

Kidney Stone Diet Recipes 18

    Skinny Banana Pudding 18

    Honey Mustard Salmon 19

    Blueberry baked oatmeal 21

    Arugula Salad 23

    Low Sodium Sloppy Joes 25

    Crispy Falafel 27

    Deb's Kale Salad with Apple, Cranberries and Pecans 30

Thai Cucumber Salad 33

Tomato & Mozzarella Salad 35

Crustless Zucchini Quiche 37

Roasted Garlicky Brussels Sprouts 39

Egg Roll in a Bowl 40

Mediterranean Chickpea Salad Bowl 42

Panzanella Toscana 45

Stir fry 47

Crispy stuffed zucchini 48

Homemade Onion Rings 50

Grilled chicken with mango avocado salsa 52

Parmesan Roasted Broccoli 53

Garlic Sauce Chicken 55

10 Minute Garlic Bok Choy Recipe 57

Chili-Lime Cod Fillets 59

Roasted butternut squash and bacon soup..... 61

Almond Pecan Caramel Corn 64

Chicken with Cornbread Stuffing 66

Beef Jerky 69

Chinese Chicken Salad 72

Collard Greens 73

40-Second Omelet 75

Cider Cream Chicken 77

Hungarian Goulash 78

Energy Bars 80

Marinated & Grilled Portobello Mushrooms 81

Honey Herb Glazed Turkey 82

Apple and Cream Cheese Torte 85

DISCLAIMER

Please note that the information and recipes in this book are written for the express purpose of sharing educational information only. The information herein is stated to be reliable and consistence, but the author neither implies nor intends any guarantee of accuracy for specific cases or individuals.

It is recommended that you consult a licensed professional before beginning any practise relating to your diet or lifestyle. The contents of this book are not replacement for professional advice.

The author, publisher and distributors disclaim any liability, loss or damage and risk taken by individuals who directly or indirectly act on the information contained in this book.

Introduction

Nephrolithiasis also known as kidney stones "are hard masses developed from crystals that separate from the urine within the urinary tract. Normally, urine contains chemical that prevent or inhibit the crystals from forming. These inhibitors do not seem to work for everyone, and stone can start to form. If crystals remain tiny enough, they will travel through the urinary tract and pass out of the body in the urine without being noticed. If the stones are unable to pass with the urine, further medical attention is needed."

Types of Kidney Stones

Calcium stones: Calcium oxalate or calcium phosphate. Calcium stones are due to high levels of calcium in the blood (hypercalcemia, hyperparathyroidism), excess filtration of calcium into the urine such as in inflammatory bowel disease, a persistent alkaline pH of the urine which enhances crystallization, or a low urine output which concentrates all stone-making elements.

Uric acid stones: From persistent hyperacidic urine (pH <5) or from uric acid overproduction and excretion.

Cystine stones: From a genetic recessive disorder (cystinuria).

Struvite stones: Magnesium ammonium phosphate stones due to infections with certain bacteria

Symptoms of Kidney Stone

You might not realize right away that you have a kidney stone. When the stone is still in your kidney, you might not feel it. If the stone is very small, it might be able to move through your urinary tract and leave your body with urine, without causing any problems.

However, when a stone travels to your ureter (tube leading from your kidney to the bladder), you will likely feel symptoms. Kidney stones are sometimes considered "the great mimicker" because their signs and symptoms are very similar to appendicitis, ovarian or testicular conditions, gastritis, and urinary tract infections. You may not feel pain in your kidneys; you may feel it elsewhere, due to pain referral patterns.

The most common signs and symptoms of kidney stones include:

- Burning during urination
- Flank pain (e.g., pain in the side of the abdomen, toward the back)
- Frequent and/or urgent urination
- Groin pain
- Nausea and vomiting
- Pain in the testicles
- Pain overlying the bladder

- Recurring urinary tract infections
- Visible or microscopic blood in the urine (hematuria)

Symptoms can be mild to severe and unrelenting. Classic kidney stone pain is often referred to as "colic," which implies that the pain comes and goes. In reality, kidney stone pain can be constant and severe and make it extremely difficult to find a comfortable position.

What Causes Kidney Stones?

There is no consensus as to why kidney stones form.

Heredity: Some people are more susceptible to forming kidney stones, and heredity may play a role. The majority of kidney stones are made of calcium, and hypercalciuria (high levels of calcium in the urine) is one risk factor. The predisposition to high levels of calcium in the urine may be passed on from generation to generation. Some rare hereditary diseases also predispose some people to form kidney stones. Examples include people with renal tubular acidosis and people with problems metabolizing a variety of chemicals including cystine (an amino acid), oxalate, (a salt of an organic acid), and uric acid (as in gout).

Geographical location: There may be a geographic predisposition to forming kidney stones, so where a person lives may make it more likely for them to form kidney stones. There are regional "stone belts," with people living in the southern United States having an increased risk of stone formation. The hot climate in this region combined with inadequate fluid intake may cause people to be relatively dehydrated, with their urine becoming more concentrated and allowing chemicals to come in closer contact to form the nidus, or beginning, of a stone.

Diet: Diet may or may not be an issue. If a person is susceptible to forming stones, then foods high in animal proteins and salt may increase the risk; however, if a person isn't susceptible to forming stones, diet probably will not change that risk.

Medications: People taking diuretics (or "water pills") and those who consume excess calcium-containing antacids can increase the amount of calcium in their urine and potentially increase their risk of forming stones. Taking excess amounts of vitamins A and D are also associated with higher levels of calcium in the urine. Patients with HIV who take the medication indinavir (Crixivan) may form indinavir stones. Other commonly prescribed medications associated with stone formation include phenytoin (Dilantin) and antibiotics like ceftriaxone (Rocephin) and ciprofloxacin (Cipro).

Underlying illnesses: Some chronic illnesses are associated with kidney stone formation, including cystic fibrosis, renal tubular acidosis, and inflammatory bowel disease.

How are kidney stones diagnosed?

Most people are diagnosed with kidney stones after the thunderclap onset of excruciating and unforgettable pain. This severe pain occurs when the kidney stone breaks loose from the place that it formed, the renal papilla, and falls into the urinary collecting system. When this happens, the stone can block the drainage of urine from the kidney, a condition known as renal colic. The pain may begin in the lower back and may move to the side or the groin. Other symptoms may include blood in the urine (hematuria), frequent or persistent urinary tract infections, urinary urgency or frequency and nausea or vomiting.

When your doctor evaluates you for a kidney stone, the first step will be a complete history and physical examination. Important information regarding current symptoms, previous stone events, medical illnesses and conditions, medications, dietary history and family history will all be collected. A physical examination will be performed to evaluate for signs of a kidney stone, such as pain in the flank, lower abdomen or groin.

Your doctor will perform a urinalysis, to look for blood or infection in the urine. A blood sample will also be collected so that kidney function and blood counts can be measured.

Even though all of these tests are necessary, a kidney stone can only be definitively diagnosed by a radiologic evaluation. In some cases, a simple X-ray, called a KUB, will be adequate to detect a stone. If your doctor requires more information, an intravenous pyelogram (IVP) or a computed tomography (CT) scan may be necessary.

Sometimes kidney stones do not cause any symptoms at all. Such painless stones can be discovered when your doctor is looking for other things on X-rays. Sometimes, although a stone does not cause any pain, it can cause other problems, such as recurring urinary tract infections or blood in the urine.

How to prevent kidney stones

There are multiple natural ways to prevent kidney stones from occurring. In some cases, dietary changes may be enough to prevent stones from occurring again. But in other cases, additional medication or surgery may be needed.

If you have passed a stone before, it is helpful to get it tested to learn what type of stones you have and what prevention tips may work best for you.

Drink lots of water: The most important thing to do to prevent kidney stones is to drink plenty of water, which helps flush compounds out of the kidneys before they can start making trouble.

Reduce sodium intake: Sodium is a natural mineral found in some foods and also makes up 40% of table salt, with chloride making up 60%. We get most of our sodium from table salt. A person with a history of kidney stones should consume less sodium/salt, because the salt in urine does not allow the calcium to be reabsorbed into the blood. This can lead to urine with high levels of calcium, which may lead to stones.

For someone whose sodium consumption has contributed to their stones in the past, I recommend reducing your sodium intake to 1,500 mg each day (one teaspoon of salt contains 2,325 mg of sodium).

When trying to have a low-sodium diet, it's important to read food labels. Foods that you should stay away from include:

- Canned soups.
- Canned vegetables.
- Chips, crackers, pretzels and other processed foods.
- Lunch meat.
- Hotdogs, bratwurst and sausages.
- Cheese.
- Condiments.
- Pickles and olives.

Foods that contain monosodium glutamate, sodium bicarbonate (baking soda) and sodium nitrate.

Eat your veggies: A diet high in fruits and vegetables, which raises the pH of the urine, can help prevent kidney stones.

Keep protein intake moderate: High protein diets, which lower the pH of your urine, can make kidney stones more likely. If you are nervous about kidney stones, you'll probably want to stick to a moderate protein diet and get at least some of your protein from plants.

Get enough calcium: A low calcium diet can also be a risk factor. This fact surprises a lot of people because kidney stones often contain a lot of calcium, which seems to suggest that too much calcium would be to blame. But it's actually the opposite. When your diet is higher in calcium, less of it is absorbed in the digestive tract and less ends up in the urine. The best way to get calcium is by eating a variety of calcium-containing foods (such as dairy products, leafy greens, tofu, canned fish) throughout the day. Taking your entire dietary allowance of calcium at one time in the form of a supplement, on the other hand, may slightly increase your risk of stones.

Limit oxalate-rich foods: Oxalate is a natural compound found in food that binds with calcium in the urine and can lead to kidney stones forming. By limiting these types of foods, you can help prevent kidney stones from forming.

Oxalate and calcium bind together in the digestive tract before reaching the kidneys. If you would like to eat foods that contain oxalate or the mineral calcium, it is best to consume them at different times.

Foods to reduce or stay away from that are high in oxalates include:

- Chocolate.
- Coffee.
- Spinach.
- Sweet potatoes.
- Rhubarb.
- Peanuts.
- Beets.
- Wheat bran.
- Almonds.

- Soy product

Kidney Stone Diet Recipes

Skinny Banana Pudding

Servings: 16

Ingredients

- 1 large box sugar-free vanilla instant pudding and pie filling mix
- 3 cups skim milk
- 2 cups vanilla nonfat Greek yogurt
- 1 (8-ounce) container light Cool-Whip
- 1 box reduced-fat Vanilla wafers
- 6 bananas, sliced

Instructions

1. In a large bowl, beat pudding mix and milk with a hand-held mixer until smooth and starting to get thick.
2. Using a rubber spatula, fold in yogurt and then Cool Whip. Set aside.
3. Place 1/3 of the Vanilla wafers in bottom of a 3-quart baking dish. Spread 1/3 of pudding mixture on top.
4. Layer 1/2 of banana slices on top of pudding.
5. Repeat layers- cookies, pudding, and bananas. Finish off with a final layer of pudding and cookies.
6. Refrigerate at least 3 hours before serving.

Honey Mustard Salmon

Servings: 4

Ingredients

- 3 Tbs white vinegar
- 1 Tbs sugar
- 3 Tbs Dijon mustard
- 1 1/2 tsp dry mustard
- 3 Tbs canola oil
- 4 4oz salmon fillets
- 1 tsp dried thyme
- 1/2 tsp black pepper
- 1/2 cup breadcrumbs

Instructions

1. Whisk together vinegar, sugar, Dijon mustard and dry mustard. Slowly whisk in oil.
2. Preheat oven to 375°F.
3. Season salmon with thyme and black pepper. Spread 1 Tbs mustard sauce

over each piece of salmon. Press breadcrumbs onto fish.
4. Place salmon on baking sheet. Bake salmon until crispy and golden brown, approximately 18 minutes.
5. Serve remaining mustard sauce on the side.

Blueberry baked oatmeal

Servings: 6

Ingredients

- 1 ½ cups rolled oats
- ½ cup milk
- 1/3 cup brown sugar
- ¼ cup melted butter
- 2 large eggs, beaten
- 1 teaspoon baking powder
- 1 teaspoon cinnamon

- 1 teaspoon vanilla extract
- ¾ teaspoon salt
- 1 cup blueberries, fresh or frozen

Instructions

1. Preheat oven to 350 degrees. Spray an 8x8 baking dish with non-stick spray.
2. Add all of the ingredients except for the blueberries to a mixing bowl and stir well to combine.
3. Fold in the blueberries gently so as not to break them up too much.
4. Spread mixture into the prepared baking dish and bake for 30 minutes or until a knife comes out mostly clean with just a few moist crumbs.
5. Spoon into bowls and serve with additional blueberries and a drizzle of cream or syrup, if desired.

Arugula Salad

Servings: 6

Ingredients

For the arugula salad:

- 5 ounces arugula about 5 cups
- 4 medium carrots shaved into ribbons (about 8 to 10 ounces) or 1 cup grated carrots (if you're in a hurry, you can use the pre-bagged grated carrots)
- 1 pint cherry tomatoes halved
- ⅓ cup large Parmesan cheese shavings see pictures—don't skip this, and the better the quality of the cheese, the better the salad! I like to shave mine right off of the block with a vegetable peeler

- 3 tablespoons chopped sunflower seeds or chopped nuts of choice—toasted and chopped walnuts pecans, and pistachios are all delicious (optional)
- 1 tablespoon chopped mild fresh herbs of choice such as chives, parsley, or tarragon (optional)

For the dressing:

- 2 tablespoons freshly squeezed lemon juice about ½ medium lemon
- 1 tablespoon balsamic vinegar
- 2 tablespoons extra-virgin olive oil
- ½ teaspoon kosher salt

Instructions

1. Place the arugula, carrots, and tomatoes in a large bowl.

2. In a small bowl or large measuring cup, whisk together the dressing ingredients: lemon juice, balsamic vinegar, olive oil, and salt. (Alternatively, you can shake them all together in a mason jar with a tight-fitting lid).
3. Drizzle enough over the arugula to moisten it, then toss to combine.
4. Sprinkle Parmesan and any desired nuts or herbs over the top. Serve immediately with a drizzle of extra dressing as desired.

Low Sodium Sloppy Joes

Servings: 6 2/3 cup

Ingredients

- 1.25 pound ground sirloin

- 2 tbsp low sodium tomato paste
- 1/2 large onion diced
- 1/2 large green bell pepper diced
- 3 cloves garlic minced
- 2 tbsp chili powder
- 2 tsp brown sugar
- 1 1/2 tsp ground mustard
- 1/8 tsp crushed red pepper flakes
- 2 tbsp apple cider vinegar
- 5 tbsp ketchup
- 1/3 cup water

Instructions

1. In a large saute pan, brown the ground sirloin. If you don't use lean ground sirloin, drain the excess fat after browning.
2. Add tomato paste and cook 1-2 minutes until tomato paste has deep

red color. Add onion, green pepper and garlic. Continue to cook 3-5 minutes until vegetables are slightly softened.
3. Add remaining ingredients. Mix well. Cover and cook 10-15 minutes.

Nutrition Facts

Nutrition Facts (per 2/3 cup): 148 calories, 10g carbohydrate, 1.6g fiber, 3.9g added sugar, 4g fat, 1.6g saturated fat, 60mg cholesterol, 19g protein, 238mg sodium, 25mg calcium, 437mg potassium, 169mg phosphorus, 5mg oxalate

Crispy Falafel

Servings: 6

Ingredients

- ¼ cup + 1 tablespoon extra-virgin olive oil
- 1 cup dried (uncooked/raw) chickpeas, rinsed, picked over and soaked for at least 4 hours and up to 24 hours in the refrigerator
- ½ cup roughly chopped red onion (about ½ small red onion)
- ½ cup packed fresh parsley (mostly leaves but small stems are ok)
- ½ cup packed fresh cilantro (mostly leaves but small stems are ok)
- 4 cloves garlic, quartered
- 1 teaspoon fine sea salt
- ½ teaspoon (about 25 twists) freshly ground black pepper
- ½ teaspoon ground cumin
- ¼ teaspoon ground cinnamon

Instructions

1. With an oven rack in the middle position, preheat oven to 375 degrees Fahrenheit. Pour ¼ cup of the olive oil into a large, rimmed baking sheet and turn until the pan is evenly coated.
2. In a food processor, combine the soaked and drained chickpeas, onion, parsley, cilantro, garlic, salt, pepper, cumin, cinnamon, and the remaining 1 tablespoon of olive oil. Process until smooth, about 1 minute.
3. Using your hands, scoop out about 2 tablespoons of the mixture at a time. Shape the falafel into small patties, about 2 inches wide and ½ inch thick. Place each falafel on your oiled pan.
4. Bake for 25 to 30 minutes, carefully flipping the falafels halfway through baking, until the falafels are deeply

golden on both sides. These falafels keep well in the refrigerator for up to 4 days, or in the freezer for several months.

Deb's Kale Salad with Apple, Cranberries and Pecans

Servings: 4

Ingredients

Salad

- ½ cup pecans
- 8 ounces kale (I used regular curly green kale, but Deb recommends Cavolo Nero or Lacinato, Dinosaur or Tuscan Kale)
- 4 to 5 medium radishes

- ½ cup dried cranberries (or dried cherries)
- 1 medium Granny Smith apple
- 2 ounces soft goat cheese, chilled

Dressing

- 3 tablespoons olive oil
- 1 ½ tablespoons apple cider vinegar (or white wine vinegar)
- 1 tablespoon smooth Dijon mustard
- 1 ½ teaspoons honey or maple syrup
- Sea salt and freshly ground pepper, to taste

Instructions

1. Preheat the oven to 350 degrees and spread the pecans on a baking tray. Toast them until lightly golden and fragrant, about 5 to 10 minutes, tossing them once or twice to make sure they

bake evenly. Remove the tray from the oven and set them aside to cool.

2. Pull the kale leaves off from the tough stems and discard the stems. Use a chef's knife to chop the kale into small, bite-sized pieces. Transfer the kale to a big salad bowl. Sprinkle a small pinch of sea salt over the kale and massage the leaves with your hands by lightly scrunching big handfuls at a time, until the leaves are darker in color and fragrant.

3. Thinly slice the radishes (this is easier to do if you first chop off the root end so you can place the base of the radish flat against your cutting board). Add them to the bowl.

4. Coarsely chop the pecans and cranberries (or cherries) and add them

to the bowl. Chop the apple into small, bite-sized pieces and add it to the bowl as well. Crumble the goat cheese over the top.

5. In a small bowl, whisk the dressing ingredients together and pour the dressing over the salad. Toss until the salad is evenly coated with dressing. Serve immediately, or for even better flavor, let the salad marinate in the dressing for 10 to 20 minutes beforehand.

Thai Cucumber Salad

Servings:5

Ingredients

- 1/3 cup rice vinegar
- 2 Tbsp sugar

- 1/2 tsp toasted sesame oil
- 1/4 tsp red pepper flakes
- 1/2 tsp salt
- 2 large cucumbers (peeled and sliced)
- 3 green onions (diced)
- 1/4 cup chopped peanuts

Instructions

1. To start, peel and slice your cucumbers long wise. Scoop out of the seeds and then slice the cucumbers. Place the cucumbers in a bowl.
2. In a small bowl, make your dressing. The Sesame Oil adds so much flavor, even though you just need a little bit. Mix together vinegar, sugar, oil, red pepper flakes and salt.

3. Pour the dressing over the cucumbers. Garnish with sliced green onions and peanuts.
4. Toss everything together.
5. Serve your Thai Cucumber Salad immediately or I personally like to let it refrigerate for a bit.

Tomato & Mozzarella Salad

Servings: 2

Ingredients

- 1/2 cup fresh cilantro
- 1 clove garlic
- 1 lime juiced
- 1 tsp honey
- 2 tbsp olive oil
- 1 pinch salt
- 6 cups romaine chopped

- 2/3 cup cherry or grape tomatoes halved
- 2/3 cup frozen corn thawed
- 1/2 avocado sliced
- 1/4 cup roasted unsalted sunflower seeds
- 2 oz fresh mozzarella sliced

Instructions

1. Make dressing. Blend cilantro, garlic, lime juice and honey in a food processor or blender until smooth. Add olive oil and blend just until combined. Season with pinch of salt. This will make about 1/3 cup dressing, enough for 2 salads.
2. To build salad, plate 3 cups lettuce, 1/3 cup tomato, 1/3 cup corn, 1/4 avocado, 2 tablespoons sunflower seeds and 2

oz fresh mozzarella. Drizzle with 2 1/2 tablespoons dressing. Enjoy!

Crustless Zucchini Quiche

Servings: 8

Ingredients

- 1 zucchini grated
- 1 small onion chopped
- 4 eggs
- 2 cups part-skim mozzarella cheese shredded
- 1 cup low-fat, reduced sodium cottage cheese
- 1 4.5oz can green chiles
- 1/2 teaspoon black pepper
- 1/4 cup green onion chopped

Instructions

1. Preheat oven to 375'F. Spray a 9-inch pie plate with cooking spray.
2. Press grated zucchini into paper towels to absorb as much liquid as possible.
3. Heat a medium skillet over medium-high heat and spray with cooking spray. Add onion and cook until softened, about 5 minutes. Add zucchini and cook until softened, about 3 minutes. Set aside.
4. In a large bowl, whisk eggs until thick and fluffy. Add mozzarella, cottage cheese, chiles, pepper and cooked zucchini mixture. Stir to combine.
5. Pour into prepared pie plate. Bake 35-40 minutes until top is puffed and golden brown and a toothpick inserted

into the center of the quiche comes out clean.

6. Garnish with green onion.

Roasted Garlicky Brussels Sprouts

Servings: 4

Ingredients

- 8 oz (about 25 sprouts) Brussels sprouts trimmed & halved
- 2 Tbs white vinegar
- 2 tsp honey
- 2 tsp Dijon mustard
- 1/8 tsp black pepper
- 1 dash salt
- 1 clove garlic minced
- 2 Tbs olive oil

Instructions

1. Place Brussels Sprouts on baking sheet. Recommended: Crowd sprouts ontoone side of sheet to prevent drying out.
2. Roast sprouts at 400°F for 20-25 minutes or until fork-tender.
3. Meanwhile, combine remaining ingredients.
4. When sprouts are done, combine with dressing.

Egg Roll in a Bowl

Servings: 6 Cups

Ingredients

- 2 tsp sesame oil divided
- 1 lb ground chicken
- 14 oz bag coleslaw mix
- 8 oz white mushrooms sliced

- 4 cloves garlic chopped & divided
- 4 green onions sliced, whites & green separated
- 2 tbsp white vinegar
- 2 tbsp low sodium soy sauce
- 1 tbsp fresh ginger grated
- 1 lime
- 1 tsp Sriracha (or your favorite hot sauce)
- 1 tsp cornstarch
- 3/4 cup fried wonton strips

Instructions

1. In a large sided skillet, heat 1 teaspoon of sesame oil over medium high heat. Add chicken and cook until browned.
2. Add coleslaw mix, mushrooms, garlic and white parts of green onion. Cook

until cabbage is tender, about 10 minutes.

3. Meanwhile, prepare sauce. Whisk vinegar, soy sauce, ginger, juice from 1/2 the lime, Sriracha and cornstarch together.
4. Add sauce to chicken & cabbage mixture. Cook 1-2 minutes, until well combined.
5. Serve garnished with sliced green parts of green onion, lime wedges and 2 tablespoons wonton strips per serving. Serve over rice if desired. Enjoy!

Mediterranean Chickpea Salad Bowl

Servings: 4

Ingredients

Mediterranean Chickpea Salad

- 15.5 oz can chickpeas, drained
- 1 cup cucumbers, diced
- 1 cup cherry tomatoes, halved
- 3/4 cup parsley leaves, diced
- 1/3 cup red onion, diced
- 1/4 cup feta crumbles

Dressing

- 2 garlic cloves, minced
- 2 tbsp lemon, juice of
- 3 tbsp olive oil
- 2 tbsp red wine vinegar
- 1/2 tsp dried oregano
- 1/2 tsp agave (can sub sugar)
- salt to taste (I used about a 1/2 tsp)

For the Bowl

- 1/2 cup quinoa, cooked, or more as needed
- 1/2 cup arugula, or more as needed
- 1 heaping spoonful roasted garlic hummus
- 1 warm pita bread, cut in triangles

Instructions

1. In a large bowl toss together chickpeas, tomatoes, cucumbers, onion, parsley, and feta.
2. Make the dressing, in a small jar whisk together minced garlic, lemon juice, olive oil, red wine vinegar, oregano, agave, and salt.
3. Pour dressing over salad and toss. Enjoy

4. To make a nourish bowl serve over quinoa and arugula. Top with hummus and warm pita bread.

Panzanella Toscana

Servings: 10 Cups

Ingredients

- 3 tablespoons olive oil
- 4 cups sourdough bread 1" cubes
- 2 large tomatoes 1" chunks
- 1 cucumber 1" chunks
- 1 red bell pepper 1" chunks
- 1 yellow bell pepper 1" chunks
- 1/2 red onion 1" chunks
- 20 fresh basil leaves roughly chopped
- 3 tablespoons capers
- 2 cloves garlic minced
- 1 teaspoon Dijon mustard

- 3 tablespoons white or red wine vinegar
- 1/2 cup olive oil
- 1/2 teaspoon black pepper

Instructions

1. Preheat oven to 375'F. Drizzle 3 tablespoons olive oil over bread cubes and place on baking sheet. Bake about 10 minutes, until bread is toasty and slightly browned. Set bread cubes aside.
2. Place tomatoes, cucumber, bell peppers, red onion, basil and capers in a large salad bowl.
3. Whisk garlic, mustard, vinegar, olive oil and black pepper together.
4. Add bread and dressing to salad bowl. Toss to combine. Let sit at least 10

minutes to allow the bread to soak up some of the dressing.

Stir fry

Servings:

Ingredients

- Precooked rice, flavored with finely chopped garlic and ginger
- 1 Red bell pepper, Julienned
- 1 small onion, slices thin
- 1 cup red cabbage, sliced
- 2 stalks celery, julienned

Instructions

1. Sauteed veggies on high in olive oil
2. Serve over rice.

Crispy stuffed zucchini

Servings:

Ingredients

- 4 large zucchini halved lengthwise
- 2/3 cup panko breadcrumbs
- 1/2 cup fresh grated parmesan cheese
- ¼ cup finely chopped parsley
- 4 cloves garlic, minced
- 1/4 cup melted butter
- Salt and pepper

Instructions

1. Preheat oven to 400°F (200°C). Spray a baking tray or sheet with non stick cooking oil spray.
2. Arrange zucchini halves, cut side up, on the baking sheet. Set aside.

3. Mix together the breadcrumbs, parmesan cheese, parsley and garlic in a small bowl.
4. Pour in the melted butter, season with ¾ teaspoon salt and ⅓ teaspoon pepper (or to taste). Mix the ingredients together until the breadcrumbs absorb the butter (about 40 seconds).
5. Spoon the mixture over each zucchini half, to evenly cover. Spray the topping with a little cooking oil spray.
6. Bake for 20 minutes in the hot oven until the crust is golden and the zucchini halves are cooked through.
7. Broil for a further 5 minutes on medium heat to crisp the topping.
8. Garnish with parsley and serve as a side accompaniment to any main dish.

Homemade Onion Rings

Servings: 2

Ingredients

- 2 large yellow onions (its all I had); cut into 1/2 slices
- 1 cup all purpose flour; divided
- 3/4 cup buttermilk
- 1 egg
- 1/2 tsp. baking powder
- 1/2 tsp. paprika
- 2 tsp. pepper; divided
- 2 – 3 Tbsp. Franks Hot Sauce
- 1 1/2 cups Panko breadcrumbs
- 1 tsp. seasoning salt
- oil for frying

Instructions

1. Using a heavy bottom frying pan - like a Cast Iron skillet, head at least 2 cups of canola oil over medium heat.
2. Set up a dredging station - I used three bowls.
3. Bowl #1 - add flour and 1 tsp pepper; set aside
4. Bowl #2 - Combine the other 1/2 cup of flour, buttermilk, egg, baking powder, paprika, salt and pepper and 2 – 3 Tbsp. of Franks Hot Sauce in a bowl and mix well.
5. Bowl #3 - add Panko breadcrumbs and seasoning salt.
6. Working in small batches, dredge the cut onion rings in the four, followed by a dip in the liquid batter and then into the Panko breadcrumbs.

7. Place in hot oil and fry until both sides are golden brown - about 3 minutes.
8. Drain off oil on and continue until all the onions are done.
9. Serve with your favorite dipping sauce.

Grilled chicken with mango avocado salsa

Servings: 4

Ingredients

- 4 thin boneless skinless chicken breasts
- 2 teaspoons olive oil
- 2 teaspoons chili powder
- salt to taste
- 1 cup diced mango
- 1 cup diced avocado
- the juice of 1 lime

- 1/2 cup minced red bell pepper
- 1/4 cup chopped cilantro

Instructions

1. Heat a grill over medium-high heat. Drizzle the olive oil over the chicken breasts and sprinkle with the chili powder and salt to taste.
2. Grill for 4-5 minutes on each side or until cooked through.
3. While the chicken is cooking, combine the mango, avocado, red bell pepper and cilantro in a bowl. Stir in the lime juice and salt to taste.
4. Spoon the salsa over the chicken and serve.

Parmesan Roasted Broccoli

Servings:5

Ingredients

- 1 pound broccoli
- 2 tablespoons oil
- ½ teaspoon garlic powder
- ¼ teaspoon salt
- ⅛ teaspoon pepper
- ½ cup parmesan cheese (shredded)

Instructions

1. Preheat oven to 400 degrees and prepare a baking sheet with nonstick cooking spray.
2. Chop broccoli and place them in a mixing bowl. Toss to coat in oil then season and toss to coat again.
3. Place broccoli on your prepared baking sheet and top with shredded parmesan cheese.

4. Bake for 25-30 minutes or until broccoli is tender.

Garlic Sauce Chicken

Servings:4

Ingredients

- 3 tablespoons olive oil
- 2 pounds chicken thighs
- salt and fresh ground pepper, to taste
- 1 whole bulb of garlic, peeled, cloves separated
- 1 cup white wine (use a wine that you like)
- 3 tablespoons chopped fresh parsley
- 1 sprig fresh rosemary

Instructions

1. Heat olive oil in a large skillet.

2. Add chicken and season with salt and pepper.
3. Cooking over medium heat, brown the chicken on both sides; about 4 minutes per side.
4. Remove chicken from skillet and set aside.
5. Add garlic cloves to the skillet and cook, stirring frequently, until golden; about 3 minutes. DO NOT BURN the garlic.
6. Carefully add wine to the skillet.
7. Stir in parsley and add rosemary.
8. Transfer chicken back to skillet.
9. Cover and continue to cook over medium-low heat for 20 minutes, turning the chicken over half way through cooking. Add 1/4-cup more

wine if it looks too dry when you go to turn over the chicken.

10. Remove from heat.
11. Transfer chicken to serving dish and spoon the garlic sauce over the chicken.
12. Serve.

10 Minute Garlic Bok Choy Recipe

Servings:6

Ingredients

- 1 tbsp vegetable oil
- 5 cloves garlic (minced)
- 2 large shallots (minced)
- 2 pounds baby bok choy (halved or quartered)
- 2 tbsp soy sauce
- 1 tsp sesame oil

- 1 tsp crushed red pepper

Instructions

1. Add the oil to a large wok or skillet over medium-high heat. Swirl to coat the entire surface of the pan. Add the garlic and shallots, stirring continuously for 1-2 minutes, or until fragrant.
2. Add the bok choy, soy sauce, and sesame oil. Toss to coat and cover. Cook for 1-2 minutes, uncover and toss, and then cover and continue to cook until bok choy is cooked to desired doneness (approximately 3-5 minutes more).
3. Sprinkle with crushed red pepper and serve immediately. Enjoy!

Chili-Lime Cod Fillets

Servings: 2

Ingredients

- 1 Teaspoon Paprika
- 1 Teaspoon Dried Parsley
- ½ Teaspoon Oregano
- ½ Teaspoon Chili Powder
- ½ Teaspoon Garlic Powder
- ¼ Teaspoon Cumin
- ¼ Teaspoon Salt
- ¼ Teaspoon Freshly Ground Black Pepper
- 1/8 Teaspoon Cayenne Pepper
- 2 Tablespoons Extra-Virgin Olive Oil, divided
- 2 Cod Fillets*
- 1 Tablespoon Unsalted Butter, or use ghee for Paleo & Whole30

- Zest and Juice of 2 Limes
- Cooked Rice, Quinoa, or Cauliflower Rice, for serving
- Your Favorite Vegetable, for serving

Instructions

1. In a small bowl combine all of the spices and mix well. Using 1 tablespoon of olive oil, brush the cod filets and then rub the filets with the spice mixture. You will use the entire rub – so make sure to coat them very well. Refrigerate the cod filets for at least 30 minutes, or up to 12 hours.
2. Preheat the oven to 450º. Place the cod filets on a foil-lined baking sheet and roast in the oven for 10-12 minutes – the fish will flake easily and be opaque throughout when it's cooked through.

3. Meanwhile in a small saucepot, melt the butter with the remaining tablespoon of olive oil. Add in the lime zest and juice and swirl the pan to mix. Serve the cod overtop of your chosen accompaniments and top with the lime butter.

Roasted butternut squash and bacon soup

Servings:6

Ingredients

- 1 butternut squash (about 3 pounds), peeled, seeded and cut in 1-inch chunks
- 1 onion, diced
- 1 red bell pepper, chopped
- 4 slices bacon, diced

- 2 tablespoons olive oil
- 2 cloves garlic, minced
- Kosher salt and freshly ground black pepper, to taste

For the soup

- 4 slices bacon, diced
- 1/2 teaspoon dried thyme
- 2 1/2 cups chicken stock, or more, to taste
- 1/4 cup crumbled goat cheese
- 2 tablespoons chopped chives

Instructions

1. Preheat oven to 400 degrees F. Lightly oil a baking sheet or coat with nonstick spray.
2. Place butternut squash, onion, bell pepper and bacon in a single layer onto the prepared baking sheet. Add

olive oil and garlic; season with salt and pepper, to taste. Gently toss to combine.

3. Place into oven and bake for 25-30 minutes, or until butternut squash is tender, stirring at halftime.*

4. Heat a large skillet over medium high heat. Add bacon and cook until brown and crispy, about 6-8 minutes. Transfer to a paper towel-lined plate.

5. Heat a large stockpot or Dutch oven over medium heat. Add butternut squash mixture and thyme, and cook, stirring occasionally, until fragrant, about 1-2 minutes; season with salt and pepper, to taste. Stir in chicken stock and puree with an immersion blender.

6. Bring to a boil; reduce heat and simmer until slightly thickened, about 5-10 minutes. If the soup is too thick, add more chicken stock as needed until desired consistency is reached.
7. Serve immediately, garnished with bacon, goat cheese and chives, if desired.

Almond Pecan Caramel Corn

Servings:10

Ingredients

- 20 cups popped popcorn or about 3/4 cup popcorn kernels
- 2 cups unblanched almonds
- 1 cup pecan halves
- 1 cup granulated sugar
- 1 cup unsalted butter

- 1/2 cup corn syrup
- pinch of cream of tartar
- 1 teaspoon baking soda

Instructions

1. In a large roasting pan, layer cooked popcorn evenly with almonds and pecans.
2. In large heavy saucepan, stir together sugar, butter, corn syrup and cream of tartar.
3. Bring to boil over medium-high heat, stirring constantly. Let boil for 5 minutes without stirring.
4. Remove from heat and stir in baking soda.
5. Pour caramel evenly over popcorn mixture, stirring to coat well.

6. Bake at 200 degrees for 1 hour, stirring every 10 minutes.

7. Let cool, stirring occasionally. Store in airtight tin for up to one week.

Chicken with Cornbread Stuffing

Servings: 4

Ingredients

- 1 tablespoon fresh parsley
- 2 tablespoons + 1 1/2 teaspoons Mrs. Dash Original Blend, divided
- 1 tablespoon Mrs. Dash Chicken Grilling Blend
- 4 (4 ounce) pieces boneless, skinless chicken breast halves
- 1 tablespoon unsalted butter
- 1 cup celery, chopped
- 1/2 cup onion, chopped

- 2 teaspoons ground sage
- 2 cups (about 7 ounces) cornbread, coarsely crumbled
- 2 cups unseasoned croutons
- 1 cup fat-free low sodium chicken broth

Instructions

Chop parsley.

1. Combine 1 tablespoon Mrs. Dash Original Blend, Mrs. Dash Chicken Grilling Blend™, parsley, mix lightly.
2. Coat chicken breasts on both sides with seasoning blend mixture.
3. Spray large non-stick skillet with non-stick cooking spray.
4. Heat skillet over medium heat until hot.

5. Add chicken breasts to skillet, cook 3 to 5 minutes on each side or until lightly brown.
6. Remove chicken breasts from skillet, set aside.
7. Preheat oven to 350 degrees.
8. Melt butter in skillet over low heat.
9. Add celery, onion, 1 tablespoon + 1 1/2 teaspoons Mrs. Dash Original Blend, sage, mixing to blend.
10. Cook over medium heat 5 to 7 minutes or until vegetables are tender.
11. Remove from heat.
12. Combine cornbread crumbs and croutons in mixing bowl.
13. Add vegetable mixture and broth, mixing to blend.

14. Spoon dressing mixture to large baking dish lightly sprayed with non-stick cooking spray.
15. Arrange chicken breasts on top of dressing mixture.
16. Cover, bake at 350 degrees 45 minutes.
17. Remove cover, continue baking 5 to 10 minutes or until chicken breast registers internal temperature of 170 degrees.
18. Garnish with celery leaves, if desired.

Beef Jerky

Servings:30

Ingredients

- 3 pounds flank steak or other lean meat

- 3/4 cup sodium reduced (lite) soy sauce
- 1/2 cup red wine
- 1/4 cup dark brown sugar
- 2 tablespoons liquid smoke
- 1 1/2 teaspoons Worcestershire sauce
- 2-3 drops Tabasco sauce
- 1 teaspoon garlic powder
- 1 teaspoon liquid pepper sauce

Instructions

1. Trim (or have the butcher trim) all fat from a 3 pound flank steak or any lean meat.
2. Cut lengthwise, with the grain, into 30 long strips.
3. Place the strips in a glass dish.
4. mix all other ingredients together and pour over the beef.

5. Cover and refrigerate for at least 5 hours or overnight.
6. When you are ready to dry the meat, remove it from the marinade.
7. If you have a dehydrator, set it for 145 degrees and dry the meat for 5-20 hours.
8. If you are using the oven, preheat to 175 degrees.
9. Put wire racks on top of baking sheets and lay the strips so they are not overlapping Bake for 10-12 hours. The beef jerky should be dry and somewhat brittle when done.
10. Store your jerky in an airtight container or plastic bag. If you are keeping it for longer than a week, store it in the freezer.

Chinese Chicken Salad

Servings: 8

Ingredients

- 2 packages ramen noodles
- 3 tablespoons, divided olive oil
- 2 tablespoons sesame seeds
- 2 cups cooked chicken or turkey, diced
- 1/2 head cabbage, shredded and chopped
- 4 green onions, diced
- 1/4 cup sugar or Splenda
- 1 tablespoon sesame oil
- 1/2 cup white wine vinegar or rice vinegar

Instructions

1. Take the ramen noodles and smash while still in the packet.

2. Open packages and remove the seasoning packets.
3. Heat 1 tablespoon olive oil in a skillet.
4. Add in the dry noodles and sesame seeds.
5. Toast until golden brown.
6. Mix chicken or turkey, cabbage, and green onions in a bowl, then add the ramen noodles and sesame seeds.
7. Blend sugar, sesame oil, 2 tablespoons olive oil, and vinegar in a separate bowl.
8. Dress the salad with the dressing.

Collard Greens

Servings:4

Ingredients

- 1 1/2 teaspoons olive oil

- 1/2 onion, chopped
- 2 teaspoons garlic, minced
- 1 large bunch collard greens, stems removed
- 1/8 teaspoon black pepper
- 1/2 teaspoon red pepper flakes
- 1 to 1 1/2 cups chicken broth, low-sodium, fat free
- 2 tablespoons vinegar

Instructions

1. Heat oil over medium heat, add onions and garlic and cook until soft (do not burn).
2. Add 1/4 of the greens and toss with onions and garlic.
3. When greens are wilted, add remaining greens in batches until all are added and wilted.

4. Mix in black pepper and red pepper flakes.
5. Add broth and bring to a boil.
6. Reduce heat and simmer for 20 minutes or until tender. The broth should be almost completely reduced.
7. Remove from heat and sprinkle with vinegar before serving.

40-Second Omelet

Servings:1

Ingredients

- 2 eggs
- 2 tablespoons water
- 1 tablespoon unsalted butter
- 1/2 cup filling (vegetables, meat, seafood)

Instructions

1. Beat together eggs and water until blended.
2. In a 10-inch omelet pan or fry pan, heat butter until just hot enough to sizzle a drop of water.
3. Pour in egg mixture. Mixture should set at edges right away. With an inverted pancake turner, carefully push cooked portions at edges toward center so uncooked portions can reach the hot pan surface. Tilt pan and move as necessary.
4. Continue until egg is set and will not flow. Fill the omelet with 1/2 cup of vegetables, meat, or seafood filling, if desired. Put filling on left side if you're right handed and the right side if you're left handed.

5. With the pancake turner, fold omelet in half. Invert onto a plate with the omelet's bottom side facing up.

Cider Cream Chicken

Servings:8

Ingredients

- 4 bone-in chicken breasts
- 2 tablespoons unsalted butter
- 3/4 cup apple cider
- 1/2 cup half and half

Instructions

1. Melt butter over medium-high heat. Add chicken and brown on both sides.
2. Add cider and reduce heat to medium; simmer for about 20 minutes.
3. Remove chicken from skillet.

4. Boil cider until reduced to about 1/4 cup.
5. Add half and half over heat; whisk until slightly thickened.
6. Pour cream sauce over chicken and serve.

Hungarian Goulash

Servings:6

Ingredients

- 2 pounds beef round steak
- 1/4 cup flour
- 1/4 cup butter or oil
- 1 1/2 cups onions, chopped
- 1 cup low sodium beef stock
- 2 teaspoons sweet paprika
- 1 tablespoon red wine or wine vinegar

Instructions

1. Cut meat into 1 inch cubes and coat with flour.
2. Heat butter or oil in heavy pot and brown meat on both sides.
3. Add onion and saute.
4. Add stock. Add more as needed. It should be thick, stew like consistency but easy to stir.
5. Cover pot.
6. Simmer the meat for 1 1/2 hours.
7. Remove meat from pot; keep warm.
8. Add paprika to stock and thicken with flour or corn starch.
9. Add wine or vinegar.
10. Serve goulash with Spaetzle or noodles and salad.

Energy Bars

Servings:8

Ingredients

- 1 cup rolled oats
- 1/2 teaspoon ground cinnamon
- 3 tablespoons unsalted peanuts, chopped
- 1/4 cup semi-sweet mini chocolate chips
- 1/3 cup shredded coconut
- 3 large eggs
- 1/3 cup applesauce
- 3 tablespoons honey

Instructions

1. Heat oven to 325 degrees. Grease a 9×9 inch pan with cooking spray.

2. In a large mixing bowl, combine oats, cinnamon, peanuts, chocolate chips and coconut.
3. Beat eggs in a small mixing bowl. Add applesauce and honey and mix well.
4. Add egg mixture to the oat mixture and mix well.
5. Press mixture evenly into bottom of the greased 9×9 pan.
6. Cook for 40 minutes. Cool, and then cut into bars.
7. May keep refrigerated in an airtight container for up to one week.

Marinated & Grilled Portobello Mushrooms

Servings:6

Ingredients

- 3 large portobello mushrooms
- 1/2 cup chopped shallots
- 1/8 cup balsamic vinegar
- 1/3 cup brown sugar
- 1/8 cup sesame oil
- 2 teaspoons lite-sodium soy sauce

Instructions

1. Wash mushrooms and set aside.
2. Mix other ingredients in a shallow baking dish and place mushrooms in marinade overnight in the refrigerator.
3. Grill mushrooms 5 minutes on each side or until darkened.
4. Mushrooms will shrink with cooking.

Honey Herb Glazed Turkey

Servings: 6-8

Ingredients

- 10-12 pounds whole turkey
- 1 onion, cut into wedges
- 2 celery stalks, whole
- 1 lemon, cut into chunks
- 1/3 cup olive oil
- 1/2 cup unsalted butter
- 2 tablespoons fresh sage leaves
- 1/3 cup fresh thyme stripped from stems (about 14 stems)
- 2 fresh bay leaves
- 2 teaspoons celery seed
- 1/4 cup honey
- 2 teaspoons lemon juice

Instructions

1. Heat oven to 350 degrees.
2. Remove neck and giblets from turkey.
3. Fill bird with onion, celery and lemon.

4. Rub skin with olive oil.
5. Put on 2 sheets of aluminum foil.
6. Cover top of bird with seperate sheet of foil, which you will remove later.
7. Seal the edges of the foil and put on a rack and roast in the oven.
8. While turkey is cooking, melt butter, chop sage and thyme leaves finely.
9. Add bay leaves, chopped herbs, and honey to butter.
10. Simmer 10 minutes, until butter is lightly browned, then remove the bay leaves.
11. When the turkey reaches 145-155 degrees, raise oven temperature to 500 degrees, remove top foil and baste turkey with honey herb mixture, every 5-10 minutes or so.

12. Using a thermometer, when the turkey reaches 160 degrees remove from oven, tent with foil and let rest 30 minutes before carving.

Apple and Cream Cheese Torte

Servings: 6-8

Ingredients

- 1/2 cup unsalted butter, softened
- 3/4 cup sugar, divided in 1/4 cups
- 1 cup flour
- 8 ounces cream cheese, softened
- 1 egg
- 1 teaspoon vanilla
- 3-4 medium apples, thinly sliced
- 1/2 teaspoon cinnamon

Instructions

1. Preheat oven to 450 degrees.
2. In a medium bowl, cream butter and 1/4 cup of sugar.
3. Blend in flour.
4. Press into a spring form pan.
5. Beat cream cheese, 1/4 cup of sugar, egg, and vanilla until smooth.
6. Spread into the spring form pan.
7. Toss apples with remaining 1/4 cup of sugar and cinnamon.
8. Arrange apples over cheese filling.
9. Bake for 10 minutes.
10. Reduce oven temperature to 400 degrees and bake for an additional 25-30 minutes until filling is firm and the apples have softened.